PSYCHOSOMATIC MEDI

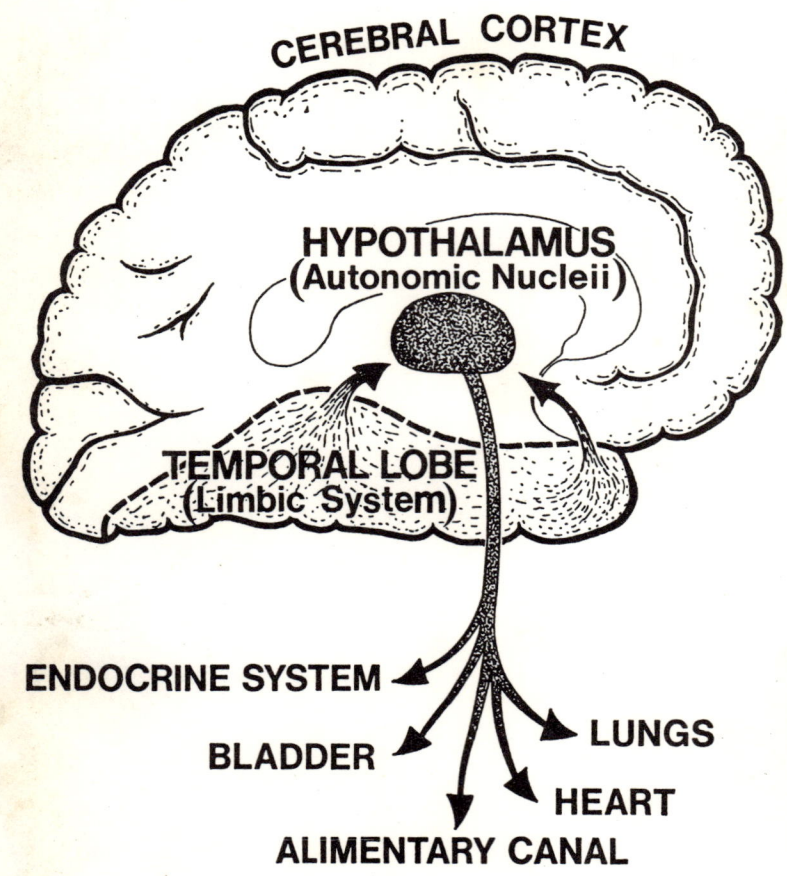

The Psychosomatic Pathways

PSYCHOSOMATIC MEDICINE FOR NURSES

Second Edition

Harold Maxwell, MD, MRCPsych
*Consultant Psychotherapist, West Middlesex
Hospital, Isleworth*

with an Introduction by

John Anderson, MD, FRCP
*Professor of Medicine, King's College Hospital Medical School,
University of London*

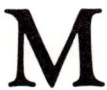

First edition published by Simon Publications (London) Ltd 1974

Second edition first published 1978 by
THE MACMILLAN PRESS LTD
London and Basingstoke
Associated Companies in Delhi Dublin
Hong Kong Johannesburg Lagos Melbourne
New York Singapore and Tokyo

Typeset by
Reproduction Drawings Ltd., Sutton, Surrey
Printed in Hong Kong

003649

British Library Cataloguing in Publication Data

Maxwell, Harold
   Psychosomatic medicine for nurses.-
   2nd ed.
   1. Nursing – Psychological aspects 2. Medicine,
   Psychosomatic
   I. Notes on psychosomatic medicine for nurses
   616.08'02'4613   RT86

   ISBN 0-333-24263-7

Contents

Preface

'. . . as you ought not to attempt to cure the eyes without the head or the head without the body so you should not treat the body without the mind.'

Socrates

The concept of whole-person, or integrated medicine is becoming of increasing importance, and practitioners in the nursing and paramedical professions (physiotherapists, opticians, radiographers, dieticians and occupational therapists) as well as physicians themselves, now fully acknowledge in their training programmes the necessity of not separating mind and body; that the uniqueness of every 'case' reflects the interaction of physical, psychological and social factors.

In this book, I have attempted to put forward views on psychosomatic disease, that is, physical illness thought to be occasioned by conflict within the mind. Frequently encountered psychosomatic conditions are discussed, with special reference to asthma and migraine, as these states exemplify, to some extent, the terms of reference under consideration; terms of reference which may be subsumed within the concept of the interrelationship of normal psychology, anxiety and body illness. At the same time, the role of nurses and ancillary workers in managing what is often a non-verbal situation, is described.

HM

Introduction

John Anderson, MD, FRCP

Professor of Medicine, King's College Hospital Medical School, University of London

As the author has suggested, it is important that all working in the medical field have a whole-person approach. This means that one cannot treat a person without knowing something about, not only the physical, but also the emotional and social sides of his illness. These are all different aspects of a person's being that make him what he is. It is all too easy to retreat into the illusion of viewing all disease as physical or on the other hand to view it all as a disturbance of the mind.

Psychosomatic diseases undoubtedly represent important areas of illness where mind and body interact in complicated ways. Perhaps some of the patterns we have come to recognise as typical of psychosomatic disease not only arise in the course of daily living but also have a background of inherited behaviour patterns. This implies that there will be both nature and nurture aspects in psychosomatic illness as well as in many other areas of medicine.

All patients, however, show interactions between mind and body when considering their own personal illness. This factor is important not only in relation to the development of illness but also in its cure. It is important for nurses and all others attending the patient to be always conscious, not only of what is spoken to them by the patient about his illness, but also of non-verbal communication. One of the tragedies is that health-care personnel often fail to notice important communications from the patient. They come at unexpected moments and are not usually elicited by direct request. I am firmly convinced that an understanding of the material presented here will make anyone who reads this book more aware of their role and provide a framework for understanding certain interesting and at times extremely difficult features of a patient's illness.

This book is recommended for consideration in the hope that it will not only benefit the reader by increasing the understanding of illness, but that it may also enable the patient to obtain from you that understanding which so many require.

1 General Definitions

Mrs R. F., aged 35, was the second of 9 children and the only one in her family to have a recurring disease since childhood: it was in fact asthma, which occurred in episodes until she was 14 and came back when her first child was 3 years old, at which time her marriage was manifestly deteriorating. After her divorce and while struggling to maintain the child on her own, no further attacks of chest trouble occurred, but subsequent to a re-marriage in her early 30s she began again to wheeze during the first trimester of her second pregnancy.

It will be apparent from this short clinical illustration that stress and anxiety may well have played a part in this patient's asthmatic episodes. Although it is a simple example it illustrates many points of what has come to be called **psychosomatic disease**, the concept of which is far from new, and which may be defined as follows:

Clinical conditions which are considered to be a compromise solution, in body terms, of emotional conflict, without initial irreversible structural changes in the organs concerned.

From biblical times the relationship between mental stress and bodily disease has been recognised. Why therefore, has it only happened in the past 25 to 30 years that psychosomatic medicine has become a speciality in its own right? Predictably the reasons are many. Perhaps one of the most important is the change in climate as to what is **'permitted'**; a notion linked with the more affluent living standard of the Western World. Hitherto people were only 'allowed' to present to doctors manifest body ailments; the idea that anything so indulgent as stress or anxiety constituted a determining factor in the aetiology was not overtly countenanced. This state of affairs obtained nowhere more than in England where the traditional stiff-upper-lip concept began even before the era of scientific medicine. Equally important have been the advances in the understanding of the anatomy and physiology of the autonomic nervous system and its connections with the various body organs, which have occurred in recent years.

Psychosomatic episodes are considered to be a temporary result of **anxiety**, the link with which may be clearly apparent, as in the case of migraine, or more hidden, as with high blood pressure. It is important to realise that psychosomatic disease is **real** disease and, as has been suggested, can eventually lead to structural changes in the organs, which may in time determine a fatal outcome. In no way may psychosomatic disease be equated with 'malingering' or with any suggestion that the sufferer is of a weaker constitution than others: it merely suggests that such a person reacts in his own way to stress which, for our purpose, results in a body disorder, as opposed to manifest mental symptoms like anxiety or depression. What has happened is that the unresolved mental conflict has become **converted** into a body symptom. The mechanism of this conversion will be considered later.

A student nurse will not be in training for long without realising the extent of psychosomatic disease. Various authors have claimed that it constitutes up to one-third of illnesses, and in some specialities, for example gynaecology, the proportion is much higher. The background to psychosomatic disease should thus be sought in the areas of ordinary human conflict to which every person is liable: broadly speaking such areas are interpersonal or intrapsychic. This simply means the factors concerned in getting on with others or with oneself. Naturally, and in very general terms, sex, occupation and social relationships are common sources of conflict, as in these situations, frustrations, slights, grudges, bitterness and above all anger and fear, are the rule rather than the exception.

It will be apparent that psychosomatic factors can be discerned in almost every illness and in order to exclude organic diseases, particularly those requiring specific therapy or surgery, the most vigorous clinical, radiological and laboratory investigations are necessary in every patient. Psychosomatic disease must in itself only be diagnosed when all other possibilities are eliminated and, as will be seen in the section dealing with affect, various criteria are sought before such a diagnosis is positively made.

2 Anatomy, Physiology and Psychology

In discussing psychosomatic disease it is necessary to consider the anatomy and physiology of the nervous system. This is divided into the central nervous system (CNS) and the autonomic nervous system (ANS). The CNS consists of the brain and spinal cord, and can be thought of as the part of the human being responsible for controlling activity and perceiving physical sensations. It is to some extent under the influence of free will and for our purpose will not be specially considered further. The ANS is composed of sympathetic and parasympathetic components, is not under the control of the will and is responsible for essential activity which is usually not conscious. It is concerned with protecting the body when the latter is confronted with any stressful situation (fright or flight). Part of the brain called the hypothalamus is linked with the ANS, and connections with the ductless glands and the viscera (internal organs) are maintained.

Sympathetic This part of the ANS is concerned with situations which threaten the individual. The emotion pertaining to it is one of fear or anger, usually both, and the **effects** come about through the activity of two hormones: adrenalin which is produced by the adrenal gland, and noradrenalin, liberated by some of the nerve endings of the sympathetic system. Adrenalin increases the heart rate and the strength of the heartbeat. It makes the heart muscle more irritable and thus predisposes it to palpitations. It leads to a rise in the blood sugar and together with noradrenalin causes the blood vessels to constrict.

Parasympathetic This system is governed by the release of acetylcholine, which substance dilates the blood vessels, causes sweating and stimulates the gastrointestinal and other internal organs to contract and secrete.

3

Mention must also be made of a more recently recognised part of the brain: the **limbic system**. This is thought to be the brain's centre of receptor-integration and anatomically consists of the hypothalamus and other proximal centres. It is thought that feelings such as frustration, rage, anger, fear and sadness are somehow transformed by the limbic centres into various body and organ effects. Probably chemicals from the limbic system mediate via the ANS, and cause changes in the internal organs of the body not controlled by the conscious will. Why this should happen in certain people more than in others is not understood: perhaps merely it is due to an innate predisposition on the part of the subject. Other patients may be in direct touch with their anger, anxiety, fear etc. and express them as such, while for our purposes the psychosomatic patient **unconsciously** denies these feelings, transforming them instead into body symptoms.

As already mentioned, among its activities the ANS stimulates the ductless or endocrine glands. These organs discharge their products directly into the bloodstream instead of via a duct into a body cavity. The pituitary, the main endocrine gland, secretes a number of hormones that influence the other endocrines, which include:

The thyroid
Sex glands
The islets of Langerhans in the pancreas
The adrenals
The parathyroids.

Diseases of the above glands are adequately described in textbooks of medicine but for the purpose of this book, the **thyroid gland** situated in the neck, merits special mention. Overactivity (thyrotoxicosis) results in some symptoms and signs very similar to anxiety states, from which careful clinical evaluation is necessary before a diagnosis is made. Sweating, anxiety, tremor and a rapid heart action will be found in both conditions, but other factors especially related to bulging of the eyes (exophthalmos) and altered levels of thyroid hormone in the blood, will point to the correct pathology. It will be noted that many of these thyroid effects are identical with those obtained by stimulation of the sympathetic system.

Hypothyroidism This not uncommon condition refers on the other hand to instances of diminished function of the thyroid gland and old people especially may be affected. Symptoms include giddiness,

4

puffiness of the skin, constipation, dryness of the hair, a generalised feeling of sluggishness and apathy, and above all, a depressive mood (see also chapter 5).

It is also important to remember the effects of body disease upon the emotions, that is the somatopsychic phenomena. Clearly any form of illness, especially that which leads a patient into hospital, will produce secondary fear, anxiety and sometimes guilt and depression. Invariably some regression in the patient's behaviour occurs, to the extent that he or she may become like a child or even a baby (see also chapter 5).

BASIC PSYCHOLOGY

'Bargains'

From the moment we are born, life presents us with problems. How to survive, and having done this, how to adapt to our environment whereby both the individual **and** the environment, which means all the people and things outside ourselves, can co-exist at a 'mutually reasonable cost'. This implies that the person and the people around him, including society as a whole, should not pay too high a price in terms of comfort and happiness in order that the individual himself may continue to function. Equally it is important that the individual himself should pay a **reasonable** price in terms of comfort for living as expediently as possible. In fact one way of looking at life as a whole is to consider whether the person and his environment can mutually adapt, so that a good 'bargain' is obtained by both. The bargain refers to the question of how the individual copes with the **inevitable** frustrations and shortcomings of life, which **cannot** be all that he expects and desires. He or the environment must adapt; must give and take. It is clear that from the start, frustrations and difficulties will beset the newborn child. He is born into a cold world having been fed and protected for nine months by his mother's body, and from which he is inauspiciously expelled. He will experience privations such as cold and hunger, and has to rely on the good will of those around him, particularly his mother, to reduce such unpleasant sensations, if indeed she cannot anticipate them. Any shortcomings on her part in this respect will constitute a source of frustration, anger and rage. Under these conditions, the baby, with its very primitive sense mechanism, will feel that it is the environment, that is, something outside itself, which is hostile, and if we can imagine tiny babies experiencing righteous anger, it can be postulated that such a state of

5

affairs may be present when a baby is left in uncomfortable conditions, like cold, hunger or wet. Thus it may be said, that from the beginning of life the environment is seen very much in terms of black and white; either it is good, that is to all intents and purposes the mother is 'good' and can adequately and quickly deal with the baby's frustrations, or she is 'bad' and neither anticipates nor speedily reduces the child's tensions, pains and discomforts. An example of this is where a baby is left to cry with hunger, or with just a wish to be held. It may seem far fetched to imagine that the baby can actually feel anger and resentment so soon after birth, but to observe babies from the first few days of life will leave no doubt in the mind of the witness that such is indeed the case. These concepts were described by Melanie Klein, a psychoanalyst working in London, who contributed in an illuminating way to infant, child and adult psychology, basing her work originally on the observation of infants and children. She postulated the useful notion that from the start of life a baby will, as has been said, split its environment (mother) into frustrating (bad) and fulfilling (good) according to whether or not the baby's needs are speedily met. Klein further thought that at this stage in life the tiny baby might find it 'easier' to indeed think of **two** mothers, one good and one bad, so that the bad one could be safely hated, leaving loving feelings which enhance development for the good, feeding mother who is always on hand and full of understanding and love. As long as this idea prevails development can take place, as in this case the bad destructive impulses and feelings could be kept discrete and not spoil the warm loving ones. As there is a natural tendency for growth and development, gradually and in normal cases, the positive instincts and attitudes will prevail.

As frustration is inevitable it will be seen how much worse the state of affairs will appear to the infant when bad mothering is actually encountered. It will then seem that the baby's worse fears are realised. In this case feeding will be irregular, and bodily concerns will neither be anticipated nor obviated for an inordinate time; a state of affairs which will enhance rage and frustration. Another analyst, Donald Winnicott, has emphasised that from the start of life it is the constancy of the mother plus her attention, which will enable development to take place naturally and positively. In terms of the psychology of development being described, it is felt that when the baby is around the age of 3-6 months, the mother starts to emerge as a **separate person**. Before this time it is thought that the newborn infant is not able to experience this, and perceives the mother merely as a collection of 'bits' and 'impressions' consisting of a source of food, warmth and physical support, and existing solely as part of the baby's needs, to the extent that the whole mother is not experienced as a separate entity. When this does occur, as mentioned above, and it becomes clear first that she **is not** merely extensions of the baby himself, development proceeds so that it is increasingly apparent that not only is she a separate individual, but she is both frustrator **and** fulfiller, that is, a good and bad mother in one.

This is a much more difficult situation to deal with. Clearly if you hate and attack the mother when she is 'bad', then because the baby in fantasy feels very powerful and dangerous (in order to make up for its real weakness), Klein believes a very frightening state of affairs develops, that is, the baby's aggressive feelings may, so it imagines, damage the bad mother who is at other times experienced as a good mother. In this way it may feel as if it jeopardises its own future as, clearly, the good, feeding, fulfilling mother must at all costs be preserved so that the baby can survive. The foregoing is a hypothesis, that is, an attempt to rationalise and explain a state of affairs which is thought to take place at a certain time in life. Undoubtedly it can be used as a useful working model from which certain phenomena common to all mankind might be explained. Klein believes that it is the solution of the above situation, that is, how to resolve the conundrum of reconciling opposing feelings towards the mother who is seen to be both good and bad, and simultaneously loved and hated, which is of the greatest importance in determining the future of the individual. It will be seen that there are many aspects in all these considerations which are governed by chance and which in no way can be attributed to the baby's idiosyncratic 'solution'. For instance, other things being equal, intelligent and experienced homes and social conditions will usually provide a better holding situation compared with less intelligent and poorer media.

For descriptive purposes one may say that the individual can make good or bad bargains with the state of affairs just described and will tend to maintain such a solution throughout his or her life. Examples of good solutions would be where gradual adaptation occurs, whereby toleration of the mother being both good and bad obtains and not **too** much is expected of her, or the future environment, or of the individual himself, so that shortcomings in all three are countenanced, and good experiences and love are stronger than frustrating and hating ones.

To reiterate, as far as the state of affairs just described is concerned, in considering the range of possible solutions and compromises, one may consider these as good or bad bargains. In the more normal state of affairs, tolerance and acceptance of the bad and good mother being one person, will lead to a gradual adaptation where love and fulfilling experiences gradually enable the individual to develop, so that a workable relationship to the environment ensues, and positive attitudes occur leading to occupations, pastimes or hobbies having at least some connotation of helpfulness or creativity. Perhaps being a member of one of the 'helping professions' may be considered as the epitome, but pastimes such as gardening or artistic creation might be seen as steps whereby the individual 'repairs' the imagined harm done to the world and those near to him when he was very small. Less desirable results would be where the obverse obtains, ambivalence is not accepted, and destructive hating impulses tend to be stronger than the loving building impulses. Here the individual's development may express itself in one of four ways:

(1) Neurotic symptoms—that is frequent anxieties, depressions, changes of mood.

(2) Psychotic symptoms. Here is meant behaviour where, unlike neurotic disorders, a greater or lesser loss of touch with reality has occurred, and there is overtly disturbed behaviour, which may range from hallucinations of sight or sound to delusions of persecution with consequent aggressive and violent manifestations. It is thought that instead of accepting ambivalence, that is the feeling of simultaneous good and bad instincts towards the same person, the individual **regresses** to a state of affairs where things are split into good and bad. Such people are suspicious, very prone to severe depressions and almost no part of their lives can develop satisfactorily.

(3) Another unsatisfactory solution might be anomalies of character and personality. Such persons may exhibit chronically difficult life styles, changing their jobs, friends, spouses and always making conditions difficult for themselves and other people. They may in addition turn to artificial means of reducing tensions such as alcohol and drugs or may even become criminals. Here both **society** and the individual have to come to terms with a bad situation.

(4) The conflict may be **converted** into a psychosomatic condition. Here mental or emotional problems are 'solved' by means of a mechanism described below; the conflict becomes what is called 'somatised', that is converted into a physical symptom and in this respect the choice of organ or part of the body in which the symptom is housed will depend on chance and on the genetic make-up of that particular person. For instance, in some families the conflict is acted out in the stomach

in terms of indigestion or peptic ulcer, while in others, the bronchi or the blood vessels of the brain (asthma and migraine respectively) will be affected.

In summary we may say that the individual's solution to ambivalence may constitute one of two **bargains**: either reasonable or bad, though it must be emphasised that there is no question of a deliberate choice— what takes place is in essence the result of the interaction of hereditary and early environmental factors.

Reasonable bargains would include an acceptable degree of neurotic anxiety and depression, appropriate especially to external situations but sometimes occurring without obvious cause, which may lead the individual to seek help or advice and even perhaps to treatment with tranquillisers or antidepressant drugs. Some form of positive living either in work and/or in hobbies will hopefully be seen as mentioned above; also one may find eccentricities of character which do not conflict with the individual's ability to earn a living or to relate to others.

Reasonable 'psychosomatic' solutions would be mild or occasional symptoms of, say indigestion, headaches, diarrhoea or asthma.

Bad bargains

(1) Neurotic, intractable depressions, or anxiety leading to chronic interference with life's enjoyments and normal pursuits, so that frequent medication or hospitalisation is necessary.

(2) Any **psychotic** solution. Here is implied a loss of the sense of reality.

(3) The character traits of anti-social behaviour perhaps leading to delinquency or even criminality. The gross recourse to drugs and alcohol. Here society pays a heavy price and makes a bad bargain, as medical care and the restraining and punitive penal systems are brought into play at considerable expense.

(4) Severe and long-standing psychosomatic conditions which lead to structural change in the organs concerned; for example heart disease, severe high blood pressure, frequent severe asthma, or ulcerative colitis.

The concept of conversion of anxiety and stress to psychosomatic disorders.

In the previous section it will have been seen that the development of personality consists of (1) normal maturation and (2) the learning to overcome the inevitable frustrations imposed by society and experienced by the whole of mankind. Thus pain, the resolution of conflicts and the experience of anxiety are, to a greater or lesser extent, mastered. With regard to the second point, one of the ways the individual does in fact achieve an amelioration of psychical pain, conflict, and frustration, is to **convert** all these unpleasant experiences into psychosomatic conditions. Exactly how this is achieved is not known, but experimental evidence suggests that the limbic system constitutes the centre whereby intolerable emotions are somehow converted into impulses generated via the ANS into the body organs.

The effects of ANS activity are the same whether the stimulation is physiological or emotional, and consist of sympathetic or parasympathetic phenomena as previously described. Generally speaking, smooth or involuntary muscle is stimulated, and sympathomimetic substances are released into the bloodstream, with secondary effects on the ductless glands producing in turn consequences on the activity of these organs.

EXAMPLES OF SUCH OCCURRENCES WITH COMMON PSYCHOSOMATIC SEQUELAE

Alterations in the calibre of the arterial blood vessels

(1) The skin vessels:	Subjective perceptions of hot and cold. Faintness. Hypotension. Skin rashes.
(2) The cerebral vessels:	Migraine.
(3) The kidney vessels:	Benign hypertension.
(4) The coronary vessels:	Chest pain on effort.

Autonomic activity affecting the sweat glands will produce secretion (sweat) and skin anomalies such as eczema and dermatitis.

Alterations in the size of the **bronchi** may result in asthma.

Overstimulation of the **vagus nerve** will often result in gastrointestinal symptoms such as indigestion, ulcer, nausea, vomiting or diarrhoea.

The bladder may 'feel' stimuli inappropriate to physiological needs, resulting in frequency of micturition.

In women, the site of anomalous stimuli may be the womb, giving gynaecological symptoms.

All the above may be acute or chronic, though the former is usually associated with situations perceived as dangerous; this may be 'real' danger, like a car skidding, so that the situation may be said to be appropriate or physiological; or originating 'in the mind' as when one meets, unexpectedly, a person with whom one has quarrelled in the past.

Chronic autonomic effects, that is those which will almost certainly result in structural changes in the organs, are those where resentment of a 'righteous' kind is felt, but for some reason is repressed, and where the state of affairs endures for a considerable time. It becomes a chronic attitude on the part of the individual which may be **transferred** from situation to situation, or from one person to another, in the person's circle of acquaintances. This repression may be at the level whereby the individual himself does not realise what or who is resented, or more commonly, where it is inexpedient, due to loyalty or fear, how to express the grievance; also in this regard, the bad circumstances may in reality be unalterable. It will be seen that 'ambivalence', a term introduced above, plays a part in these factors; examples are legion and are part and parcel of modern life. The traffic, inflation, income tax, and all the stresses of urban living may cause reasonable stress, but their effects are not considered as particularly damaging to the individual, because they are shared by all, and it is more than legitimate to grumble at them. The situations causing insidious psychosomatic manifestations are those in which the individual feels particularly ill-dealt with by fate, in a way in which he or she feels especially singled-out, and which it is difficult to alter without relinquishing something else which is felt to be needed (again the 'bargain' concept).

Situations of potential stress

Common examples include long-standing frustration due to exploitation by someone who is at once needed or even loved, such as an employer, friend or spouse. Suppressed hostility may similarly result from a snub perpetrated by a figure of authority, or those who enjoy what is felt to be a higher social status. Very often this jealously is 'projected' on to other people who then seem to threaten the individual, and thus come to share with him a mutual ill-defined antagonism.

Yet another frequently occurring source of frustration is, of course, not experiencing sufficient sexual fulfilment of the type the individual needs.

11

All these situations have in common a wound to the individual's self-esteem, dignity and pride, resulting in hostility which for our purpose becomes converted to a psychosomatic disease, as opposed to the conversion to neurotic depression or anxiety, to psychotic symptoms, or delinquent behaviour. Because of innate or acquired circumstances, certain people are particularly sensitive or vulnerable, and somehow find themselves holding grudges, possessed of inordinate envy, and appear to smoulder at life and at the people close to them especially in the spheres highlighted above. Aggression, other persons', but especially their own, both because it seems to be of tremendous strength, and also because so often the object of the anger is someone close, who is at the same time loved, valued and needed, is often repressed or purposely not expressed and may be deflected on to someone outside the acquaintance-group (vehicles for this anger are readily found in strangers, certain political or racial groups or foreigners) or, as is the theme of this book, converted into a body disease.

We have seen that individuals seem to 'choose' which organ or organ symptoms they will use. This is partly hereditary but is otherwise not well understood. Why **should** this conversion of mental anguish and pain be converted into body disease? It will be apparent that to do so may result in an 'easier' solution, at any rate on the surface. When the source of the anxiety is not well understood or when it is concerned with anger and rage, particularly towards one who is at the same time loved, the ideal solution is impossible, as opposing conditions would both need to be satisfied: clearly an intolerable state of affairs, and one not readily verbalised. In such cases it will be seen that it is much easier and 'respectable' to present oneself physically ill with, say, indigestion, high blood pressure or asthma. It may also be 'easier' than excessive changes of mood, as the individual can thus stay on better terms with his workmates and relatives, and a state of affairs is constructed, wherein as a result of body illness, he is not censured, he may be looked after, and to some extent will be enabled to dominate his environment. There is also clearly no ambivalence to the illness itself. If one has a headache there can be no doubt that one wishes it to go, and a sufferer from asthma is in no doubt as to his attitudes towards his dyspnoea. It is clear that a further way of dealing with frustration and anxiety is to experience them in a purer form such as overt anxiety and/or depression. These, of course, are not psychosomatic diseases and will be treated appropriately by the patient himself, his G.P., or a psychiatrist.

3 Systematised Psychosomatic Disease

In this section some of the conditions thought to be psychosomatic in background, will be examined. Their clinical features and medical management will be detailed only in so far as to remind the reader of the diseases as a whole, as they are fully described in general textbooks of medicine. What will be highlighted here is their special psychosomatic features as regards aetiology, general description and treatment. Asthma and migraine which are common conditions exemplifying, in the opinion of most authorities, psychosomatic disease, will be discussed more fully. Other conditions are alluded to under the following sections:

Gynaecology and Obstetrics
Cardiovascular
Pulmonary
Gastrointestinal
The Skin
The CNS

GYNAECOLOGY AND OBSTETRICS

It will be quite apparent that of all the specialities, gynaecology has very special psychosomatic overtones and meanings, and it is thought that a high proportion of conditions labelled gynaecological are expressions of a woman's conflict towards her femininity and sexuality.

13

The menstrual flow, be it regular or irregular, heavy, scanty or absent will have special significance to the patient. In physical terms the manifest bleeding comes to represent the essential 'womanliness' of a woman and whether she is happy and contented, angry or fearful, can be expressed in these variables of the monthly bleeding. Naturally this is not to suggest that they are under **conscious** control, but at a deep level, unconscious attitudes and feelings can usually be discerned when one takes a careful menstrual history, especially evaluating the presence and severity of **pain** (dysmenorrhoea).

Menstrual disorders

These will include excessive loss, too frequent periods as well as too sparse a loss and too infrequent periods, all of which are often encountered. Dysmenorrhoea, that is, painful periods, may have a somatic as well as a psychological basis, and of all gynaecological symptoms is the one *par excellence* which exemplifies the 'female protest'.

Premenstrual tension

Here especially, emotional factors are considered to be of the greatest importance. Various attitudes, which may themselves be mutually conflicting, will appear and influence the patient at different times in the menstrual cycle. During the days preceding the onset of the bleeding, changes of mood, irritability, depressions and a tendency to impulsive and contrary behaviour may be seen. Physiological causes are of the greatest importance in the production of the symptoms: essentially, this means alterations in the balance of female hormones in the blood. The mood or psychological symptoms which are no doubt produced by the foregoing, will take the form of unconscious 'reminders' of the many ambivalent attitudes and feelings that the female patient has towards her own sense of being a woman. These will include, often forgotten states of despair at not being a man, with all the imagined 'freedom' that would give her, as well as unconscious regret that pregnancy will not, at least this month, occur. This concept is linked with a view held by some schools of psychology, that at an unconscious level a pregnancy is **always** at least partly wished for, in order to repair imaginary damage done to the patient's own mother which occurred magically, when the patient was angry with the mother in the past. The situation regarding oral contraception is discussed below in this regard.

Naturally, the very realistic and proper need to avoid pregnancy is equally a factor to be taken into account: what is considered important in the production of the symptom is the unconscious conflict played out in the arena of the premenstrual situation.

The whole ambivalent process may make for tension and exasperation especially displayed towards the male partner, who it is felt gets off 'scot-free'. At the same time the period itself constitutes the instrument whereby a woman's ultimate feminity, that is motherhood, is manifested. It is known that the incidence of other illnesses, as well as a tendency towards accidents, is increased during the premenstrual phase. Physiological factors such as water-retention may also occur with secondary feelings of fullness and bloatedness.

Dysmenorrhoea

Both men and women envy characteristics of the opposite sex, and the earlier psychoanalysts, including Freud himself, thought that the initial reaction on discovering that one is a woman rather than a man is frequently one of anger and disappointment, even on the part of the youngest female child. This attitude, it is believed, persists to some extent throughout life, and the onset of the periods serves to accentuate and worsen this sense of disappointment, an attitude which colours many women's life-attitudes, determining such characteristics as moodiness, irritability, competitiveness, as well as joy and happiness in being a wife and mother. In the sexual sphere hidden anger towards men may show itself as conscious or unconscious frigidity; the latter being exemplified by vaginismus, a spasm of the muscles of the thighs and thus of the vagina so that intercourse is difficult or impossible. Fears and guilt of the sexual function consequent upon masturbation in childhood or adulthood may also have effects on the total personality as well as producing gynaecological illnesses. Thus it is thought that tension and resentment, often cryptic, is transformed into muscular over-tensions of the uterus and cervix.

Amenorrhoea

This, the stoppage or absence of the menstrual discharge, is particularly common among young women and not infrequently seen in nurses and students, especially when they first leave home. It may appear alongside episodes of depression or anxiety, especially associated with relationships, where again ambivalent feelings towards parenthood are in evidence. It may also be part of other functional diseases such as anorexia nervosa and, of course, occurs in organic states particularly associated with disorders of the endocrine glands.

Hypo-fertility

There is a well-known strange phenomenon whereby a couple may not be able to produce children over many years, following an adoption, the woman becomes pregnant. Investigations in such cases have shown a healthy feminine pelvic state of affairs throughout, while the husband's seminal count has also been normal. This strongly suggests that such a state is compounded of emotional factors mostly on the part of the woman. It may coincide with episodes of overt anxiety and depression.

Frigidity means an absence, or low level of sexual feeling when it comes to actual intercourse. Anticipatory excitement may be present to a normal degree but attempt at penetration results in a dry vulval reaction or vaginismus (spasm of the adductor muscles of the thigh and of the vagina itself). The absence of orgasm is relatively common and many women appear to be not too bothered by this fact. Parodoxically, it is often the wish to be physically held and loved by their husbands which seems to mean more to them than actual sexual climaxes. This state of affairs although accepted philosophically, nevertheless does point to a deep-seated aversion, fear or anger, towards the male partner: in fact what is happening, is that the tender, that is the 'feminine' part of the husband is being responded to. Many married couples settle for this state of affairs and a more or less successful relationship ensues.

Oral contraception

It is not too much to say that during recent years, the development of this form of family planning has revolutionised society. No longer need any woman fear an unwanted pregnancy and for the first time it is she, rather than the man, who may control this fact. While it has increased her freedom of choice and sexual life generally, a price has inevitably been paid by individual women both in physical terms (in that endocrine changes have been artifically induced with occasional hazardous results), but equally important, factors stemming from guilt have made themselves felt in the woman's own life, particularly in relationship to men.

16

She has usurped the 'male prerogative' of deciding whether or not
pregnancy may occur and has had to take the responsibility for this
fact. All the points mentioned above with regard to premenstrual tension, together with the fact that pregnancy is a monthly 'non-event',
will obtain, often to a higher degree in women on the pill, although, of
course, it must be conceded that for the first time there is the possibility
of sexuality without anxiety in the many situations where pregnancy
would be realistically undesirable. Paradoxically the taking of the oral
contraceptive may highlight sexual inadequacy on the part of the
husband, and thus cause the marriage to founder. All in all we may
expect a high incidence of anxiety and depression to be seen in women
practising oral contraception, or it may be truer to say that factors
involving ambivalence towards femininity and sex will become exaggerated.

The menopause

Usually in the mid or late 40s menstrual activity ceases and may be
accompanied by various mood manifestations which can be of almost
any type: irritability, depression, over-activity of thoughts with or
without accompanying body symptoms such as sweating or palpitations.
Almost any phenomenon seen in women of this age is usually attributed
to 'the change of life'. Naturally the implications will differ from
woman to woman with the cessation of active reproductive life. Relief,
regret, recriminations may all occur at various times. At its best it is a
time heralding an increased tranquillity, and at its worst it is the beginning of years of varying agitation. The previous personality will usually
be the best barometer to what is in store.

Thus it will be seen that many gynaecological conditions, like all
physical diseases generally, have possible emotional counterparts, and the
nurse with her special sensitivity will be able to gauge the degree of each
component when caring for women with these afflictions. Indeed she is
at an advantage compared with male **doctors** who cannot experience
similar situations, and thus are unable to fully understand and sym-
pathise with the patient.

Obstetrics

Though the normal married woman feels mostly joy at the idea of being
pregnant, at the same time she may to a greater or lesser extent exper-

17

ience at the best, misgivings and at the worst, profound misery when in this state. Indeed the latter is so common after delivery that puerperal depressions are a well-recognised clinical entity. The background of these varies considerably. On the one hand a woman's first pregnancy will realistically present her with problems mostly bound up with unknown factors, and advice and encouragement will quickly allay these real fears which are the result of lack of knowledge. Where do the other anxieties and depressive states come from? It is thought that they are associated with unconscious states of guilt at having indulged in sex so that she is now forced to show her shame to the world (and especially to her own mother). The guilt may extend to doubts about her ability, or 'right' to function as a woman, and that everything inside her is dirty and undesirable. She thus may fear that the baby will be born deformed or somehow unattractive. Alternatively, she may feel well during the pregnancy, but the puerperal depression already referred to, may ensue and here there is probably a complicated mental state whereby the women feels that all is well as long as the baby is inside her but once she has parted contact with it, she is left cold, empty and dead, for this is how she feels inside. Antidepressant drugs and relatively superficial psychotherapy usually help the condition.

THE CARDIOVASCULAR SYSTEM

Cardiovascular symptoms

Palpitations

This means an undue awareness of one's heart beat and the impression that some beats are extra forceful, irregular or 'missing'. There may be associated breathlessness, or pain in the chest, the latter of an aching character and usually distinguished from the pain of coronary disease. The cause is an increased irritability in some part of the heart or its conducting mechanism that may be brought on by external factors such as certain foods (especially those containing caffeine), undue exercise or anxiety. Alone, palpitations have no undue significance and usually the condition abates when the patient's current anxiety resolves.

Mrs H. B., aged 38, married with three children, worked as a florist and a school cleaner as well as housewife and mother. Her palpitations were present for four years. She was the fourth of five children,

18

her father having died when she was 14 and her mother when she was 33. The latter's cause of death was a heart attack. It had never occurred to Mrs H. B. to correlate her mother's fatal illness with her own present symptoms. She was a very anxious, over-active woman who 'must always do something', just 'cannot do nothing'.

Hypertension and Coronary Disease

This means blood pressure persistently higher than the normal average reading of 120 mmHg systolic and 80 mmHg diastolic. The doctor when taking these readings makes due allowance for the patient's age, sex, weight and state of mind. The figures referred to apply to the average resting readings in a subject of average weight for his given age and sex. Once again over-activity of the sympathetic system will cause the peripheral vessels to constrict and thus the heart will need to beat at a greater pressure to drive the blood around the body. Concomitant with this, the coronary vessels also constrict and thus the heart muscle's own blood supply will be impeded. If this state of affairs occurs too frequently, the reduced blood supply to the kidneys will eventually produce an additional pressor substance which in turn exacerbates the whole condition.

Mr O., aged 53, came into hospital with his second attack of coronary thrombosis. He was hypertensive (B.P. 150/95) and smoked 30 cigarettes a day. He had worked in the Colonial Service, where he was able to exercise a great deal of authority and power and had not hesitated to use corporal punishment when the opportunity presented itself. On returning to England at the age of 47 he was forced to take a relatively minor post in local government and became increasingly morose, moody and bitter at his lower status and self-esteem. His first attack of coronary thrombosis occurred soon afterwards, just after his daughter's engagement. This man invariably made the doctor feel 'uneasy': somehow the patient's cruel streak seemed always very near the surface and the symptoms were reported in a peculiarly clipped quietly smouldering tone.

Here, resentment towards the changed environment and difficulties in adaptation to circumstances less under his own control, resulted in this patient 'stifling' overt angry feelings, which became transformed via his ANS, to his skin and coronary vessels.

PULMONARY SYSTEM

Asthma

Mrs L., aged 19, the youngest of three children, was re-housed soon after her marriage, and came to live in a 'new town' many miles from her parents. Having successfully escaped much in the way of serious illness up to this time, the new experience of marriage and separation, especially from her mother, were too much for her and asthmatic attacks became established during the first year of married life. It is probable that these two factors were necessary, that is marriage and *maternal separation, for the condition to evolve. Asthma was 'chosen' as Mrs L's stress-disease probably because of its being carried in the family from a maternal grandmother. She came to find adequate support in her new husband and gradually adapted to the change of environment with a diminution in frequency and severity of her attacks.*

Of all diseases acknowledged by both the medical profession and the general public to be emotionally determined, asthma consists of episodes of **dyspnoea**, having the character of a **wheeze**. This musical breathing is due to construction on the part of the smaller bronchi which are in turn affected by changes in stimulae propagated by the ANS. As well as actual constriction on the part of the smaller tubes, their lining becomes swollen by mucosal dilation and secretion.

Diagnosis

It must be distinguished from 'cardiac asthma' which is due to left heart failure, and also from obstruction of the trachea or main bronchus due to a tumour or foreign body, in which case the stridor (deep sound) which is present, easily distinguishes this condition from the wheeze of bronchial asthma which is a high sound.

Course and prognosis

The disease often starts in infancy or childhood, is frequently accompanied by bronchitis and usually tends to improve as the individual gets older. Treatment of the attacks themselves and the general management of the patient and his environment is rewarding to the nurse and can do much for the sufferer.

Features of Asthma

Role of allergy.
Role of infection.
Clinical features.
Physical signs.
X-ray.

Role of allergy, a term meaning altered reaction. This is undoubtedly a factor in some cases where hay fever or skin rashes may co-exist or alternate with the asthma. Common foreign substances which may produce these clinical states include **inhalants**, for example pollens, feathers, moulds, and **ingestants** such as chocolate, potato, eggs, milk. Usually skin tests will establish a positive diagnosis of allergy to these substances.

Role of infection. Bronchitis, that is an infection of the bronchi due to bacteria or viruses may, as a result of secondary allergy, produce an asthmatic attack while conversely, primary, non-infective asthma may lead to the bronchi becoming infected giving **secondary** bronchitis.

Clinical features

Asthma sufferers may be of any age. The attacks can occur with sudden or gradual onset so that the patient becomes breathless, and the respiratory noises are much more audible than usual, having a characteristic high-pitched wheeze. Self-relief is attempted by the sufferer adopting an upright posture, flexing the shoulder girdle so that the accessory muscles of respiration may be exploited. Cough is a common accompaniment and this may herald the onset of an attack. The duration can vary from minutes to hours or even days when the term **status asthmaticus** is used. Eosinophil cells may appear in the sputum and blood.

Physical signs

During the paroxysm the chest is held in inspiration and the breath sounds are masked by high-pitched musical noises, especially pronounced in expiration.

X-ray shows no abnormality except in long-standing cases, when lungs may become large and ballooned (emphysematous) due to the loss of elasticity on the part of lung tissue.

Treatment

In acute asthma the patient will take up his most comfortable position, usually propped up in bed or sitting in a chair. Oxygen should be given if there is cyanosis, and antibiotics in the event of infection.

Sympathomimetic drugs may be used first. In mild cases the oral administration of ephedrine, 30–60 mg, or the inhalation of a 1 per cent solution of isoprenaline sulphate in the form of an aerosol produced by a hand nebuliser, may be sufficient to abort or arrest a paroxysm. In more severe cases a subcutaneous injection of adrenalin, 1:1000 solution, is needed. An injection of 0.5 ml, repeated if necessary 30 minutes later, should be sufficient. In some cases the patient may be taught to administer this himself. One 20 mg tablet of isoprenaline sulphate (Neo-epinine), sucked till it dissolves, is sometimes as effective as an adrenalin injection in arresting a paroxysm. The earlier these drugs are given in an attack the more effective they are.

In more severe cases intravenous aminophylline or corticosteroids are used. Morphine is never given because of its depressant effects on respiration.

Aerosols   This form of preparation is now frequently used in the treatment of asthma. It may take the form of bronchodilator drugs, such as isoprenaline, for example Medihalor, or salbutamol, for example Ventolin, the latter having a lesser side effect on the heart.

Prophylactic therapy

Where sympathomimetic drugs, orally or by aerosol, fail to provide adequate relief, prophylactic treatment with sodium cromoglycate (Intal) may be instituted. Unlike aerosol preparations this substance is not delivered under pressure, but, by means of a special device (the Spinhaler), enters the lung by the patient's own inspiratory effort. It acts by inhibiting the release of spasmogens and inflammatory agents in immediate-type allergic reactions in the lung; protection in delayed-type reactions has also been demonstrated. Controlled trials show that sodium cromoglycate offers a valuable contribution to asthma therapy. The benefits reported have included a reduction in the severity and frequency of acute attacks, especially nocturnal attacks, and reduced cough and sputum volume. Improvements in exercise tolerance and in lung function, particularly in the younger age group, frequently occur; control of exercise-induced asthma has also been reported. In addition, older patients sometimes have an unsuspected allergic element to their disease; thus trial of Intal in this upper age group is also justified. A reduction in bronchodilator usage and corticosteroid requirement has also been reported. Sodium cromoglycate has no bronchodilator or anti-inflammatory activity.

Should Intal fail to control symptoms completely, the use of oral corticosteroids may then be necessary. Corticosteroids may be prescribed in the form of an aerosol and here the amelioration in symptoms is brought about by the anti-inflammatory activity of the preparation, for example beclomethasone (Becotide) or betamethasone (Bestesol).

As with all psychosomatic conditions it may also be necessary to administer antidepressants, tranquillisers and psychotherapy (see chapter 6).

Summary

As with other psychosomatic conditions, asthma is a reflection of bad adaptation to various determinants, both internal and external. The site of this mal-adaptation, in this case the bronchi, is governed by genetic factors. Through its very nature, asthmatic subjects experience **constriction**; that is the sufferers feel shut in and claustrophobic. The allergic factor is probably conditioned by the specific inhalant or food to which the subject was originally exposed at a time when he was under some form of stress.

The effect of the severe asthmatic attack upon the environment is frightening, and engenders a state of helplessness and urgent compulsion to help. As with all psychosomatic diseases the sufferer has a 'secondary gain' from the condition; that is the environment may become dominated by him, and relatives and friends could find their attitude and behaviour to the patient altering both during and between attacks.

As asthma is so common in children, the mother–child relationship is especially important in this disease. It is easy and indeed reasonable for a mother to feel anxious, guilty, constrained and helpless because of the condition, but she must whenever possible maintain a demeanour of calm confidence, knowing realistically that a given paroxysm is almost never fatal.

Case report of childhood asthma:

B. B., aged 8. One brother 6 years older than himself. Began having asthma attacks following the birth of a sister. There was overt dismay when she first appeared, episodes of rage and frustration at

23

having to relinquish so much of his mother's time and attention. Laboured and wheezing breathing soon became apparent, which was managed sensibly by both the G.P. and the parents over the course of the next five to six years, when the episodes gradually became less severe.

GASTROINTESTINAL CONDITIONS

Common psychosomatic **symptoms** include:

Nausea, anorexia, dysphagia, 'indigestion', diarrhoea and vomiting.

Diseases of probable psychosomatic origin include:

Anorexia nervosa   Irritable bowel syndrome
Peptic ulcer   Ulcerative colitis

Nausea and anorexia

These common phenomena may occur at meal times, or merely at the thought of food, so that **anorexia** may be present to a greater or lesser degree. A severe state of the latter called **anorexia nervosa** is a not uncommon condition and is especially seen in adolescent girls. This can be a most severe and dangerous condition and is often difficult to treat. The subject at first rationalises that to take too much food is unwholesome, and that it may lead her to undue obesity giving her an ugly body-image. Alternatively, she may merely experience a deep lack of interest in food without being able to explain the reason. The emaciation and especially the low body vitamin and mineral levels make the condition, as has been stated, a highly dangerous one. Anorexia nervosa, unlike many of the psychosomatic states, is not due to over-activity of the sympathetic nervous system, but is a body reflection of a severe personality disorder.

Diarrhoea, vomiting and dysphagia

These symptoms are perhaps among the most commonly accepted by both the medical and nursing professions, as well as the general public, as being produced by anxiety, conflict and emotional upset. Nevertheless, their persistence always calls for a thorough examination, so that organic illness is not overlooked. Nervous diarrhoea which may be associated with abdominal pain is also called the **irritable bowel syndrome.**

Mrs W. B., aged 53, a widow for 12 years, came complaining of four weeks' diarrhoea and vomiting which tests had shown to be non-infective. She was one of 11 children, had two married daughters and one son aged 17 who very recently had decided to join the Army. She stated how often this boy and herself had indulged in rows and misunderstanding and how she had been taken unawares by his precipitate decision to leave home. A favourite brother had also recently died. She had been unable to see any possible link between these events and the onset of her gastrointestinal symptoms, but when the probable correlation was pointed out she did agree that possibly they had something to do with it.

The expulsion both 'upwards and downwards' reflected her difficulty in retaining the feelings associated with the double loss; the brother and the son.

Peptic ulcer

This can be oesophageal, gastric or duodenal and is dependent for its production on the interaction of peptic juice with the mucosal lining of the lower part of the oesophagus, the stomach or the duodenum. It is usually (but not always) found that patients with these conditions are overtly tense, and as a result of their genetic make-up, their anxiety 'goes to their stomach'.

Oesophagitis or **peptic ulcer** in the lower part of the oesophagus, gives rise to the symptom of heartburn and an acid taste in the mouth. With **gastric ulcer** the pain is in the epigastrium, occurs soon after eating and is made worse by food. **Duodenal ulcer** classically is felt up to 1-2 hours after meals and is relieved by the taking of more food. Nausea and occasional vomiting may be present and there is usually a disturbance of the appetite in all three conditions. The treatment is by medical or surgical means; the former being reinforced by psychotherapy, usually of a minor degree.

Ulcerative colitis

This is a not uncommon condition the cause of which is unknown, but in recent years has come to be regarded as a psychosomatic auto-immune disease. The salient symptom is bloody diarrhoea with debilitation, loss of weight and sooner or later serious metabolic disturbances.

Mrs T. M., aged 23, recently married, began having episodes of frequent blood-stained motions at puberty. She had one brother three years her senior who had achieved considerable success both academically and as an athlete. It had become established that her behaviour grew increasingly 'difficult' on first attending school and it seemed that she had never really settled down or accepted life on its own terms. There was extreme overt rivalry with the brother throughout her life and her adolescence was particularly difficult for all concerned. The attacks of colitis became rather worse after her marriage but were controlled to some extent with tranquillisers and enemas of steroids.

It is often felt that the onset of the condition follows a psychological stress though this is by no means always the case. Mild degrees of the condition often respond to steroids which may be prescribed topically in the form of enemas; severe forms of ulcerative colitis may eventually need an ileostomy, in itself a traumatic and disturbing experience with predictably, somatopsychic sequelae. While many studies have purported to show a special type of personality prone to develop ulcerative colitis, none has been conclusive and it is quite clear that the passage of frequent watery motions and blood through the rectum, would be expected to produce secondary effects on the personality. Anxiety, depression and limitation of life's activities, including the ability to earn a living and the enjoyment of social relationships, ensue, so that the colitis personality could be seen to be the result of the background of the disease. The condition is not uncommon in young people and should an ileostomy be required it will, as has been suggested, lead to emotional problems because of the risk of incontinence, although with modern toilet appliances these may be minimised. The possibility of lessening the sense of resulting isolation by means such as joining the Ileostomy Association may help the patient. One fear of subjects with ileostomies is that their sexual function will become impeded. This is usually not borne out in fact, but again sympathetic handling by doctor and nurse will do much to mitigate the risk of such an eventuality.

Chronic constipation, an endemic disease of our time due to faulty foods and anxiety-states, often leads to ano-rectal disorders such as piles, fissures and prolapse.

THE SKIN

This organ represents the boundary between the person and the world
and it is therefore not surprising that it will reflect many of the subject's
innermost feelings towards the external environment. Emotional conflicts may be mirrored in the skin, as exemplified by itching and the
predisposition to the dermatological conditions with the many titles
that skin specialists use to describe them. Such names are:

Dermatitis, Eczema, Urticaria, Rosacea, Psoriasis, Acne

A skin disease, like any other illness, affects the psyche, but on many
occasions it will be apparent that the particular case under review contains a predominant emotional factor contributing to its background. It
is thought that as with other psychosomatic conditions, the damming
up of feelings may be the fundamental cause of any disturbance of
mind or body and repressive drives may be expressed in terms of skin
disease. Of particular importance is the fact that the organ is an
erogenous zone, that is a source of pleasure or pain, and as develop-
mentally it comes from the same embryonic source as the hair and the
teeth, three organs which are all 'on view' it will be apparent that
anomalies in these parts of the body may have special significance with
regard to the individual's self-esteem, attractiveness and general sense
of well-being.

*Mr G. S., aged 47, is employed as a painter and decorator, married
with one son aged 13. He was the youngest of four children and
there had been no family history of skin trouble. His own various
dermatological states began 20 years previously when he had been
called up for National Service and for the first time was forced to
live away from home. Any minor bouts of worry or family crisis
exacerbates his eczema, which also had an 'external' determinant
in so far as he was constantly being exposed to skin irritants in his
work.*

THE CENTRAL NERVOUS SYSTEM

Epilepsy

A fully fledged fit, or attack of **Grand mal** is a dramatic occurrence.
Petit mal, though not associated with the violent body manifestations,
can be equally terrifying for the subject. Both states may be primary,

27

or secondary to some condition within the brain such as a tumour, injury or vascular anomaly. When it is primary, that is when no physical cause can be found as a result of investigations such as X-ray or exploratory operation, then the condition is said to be 'idiopathic'. The diagnosis may be confirmed by the electroencephalogram which may shown altered electrical activity within the brain, this state of affairs obtaining whether the epilepsy is primary or secondary. Psychosomatic and emotional aspects of epilepsy are well recognised, as either forms of the condition can be provoked by fatigue, anxiety or traumatic events. Untreated epilepsy is so frightening for both the patient and witnesses, and so dangerous in that the subject is unable to control his activity, that it is of the utmost importance to bring the fits under control with drugs; luckily this is usually possible. As with all conditions described in this book the **patient** with epilepsy must be treated, rather than just the epileptic attacks. An attitude of reassurance and calm as well as an overall optimistic demeanour coupled with an understanding of the patient's total life situation, will always be of paramount importance, and no-one has a more important role to play in this regard than the nurse.

Migraine

Of all the psychosomatic diseases appertaining to the CNS **migraine** is the most firmly described as such.

What is meant by migraine?

A patient will often talk about his 'migraine' rather than his headaches. The expression implies a special type of headache, though some authors believe that **any** series of recurrent headaches in one individual may be called 'migraine', and that at different times in the life of that person such an episodic head pain may be accompanied by phenomena like vomiting in childhood, spots before the eyes in adult life, etc.

A description by Gowers in 1888 includes most of the features now accepted in the establishment of the diagnosis. He wrote:

Migraine is an affection characterised by paroxysmal nervous disturbance, of which headache is the most constant element. The pain is seldom absent and may exist alone, but it is commonly accompanied by nausea and vomiting, and it is often preceded by some sensory disturbance, especially by some disorder of the sense of sight. The symptoms are frequently one sided, and from this character of the headache the name is derived, the Greek 'hemicrania' (still often employed) furnishing the French 'migraine', the German 'migran', and the English 'megrim'.

One could perhaps add that the headaches are now thought to be due to changes in the calibre of the intra- and extracranial arteries. As a corollary they are often, but not always, sensitive to ergotamine, and a diuresis of obscure origin may occur as the attack is waning.

Earliest accounts of headache do not attempt to differentiate between various types, and descriptions are given which could clearly be applied to those occasioned by toxaemias, sinusitis, trigeminal neuralgia, brain tumours and various other forms of head pain.

The nature of migraine

In considering first the incidence of the condition, the clinician must decide upon his criteria of diagnosis. Headaches, *per se*, are extremely common, and are usually dealt with by the patient himself. If concomitant features such as teichopsiae, vomiting or unilaterality of the pain are looked for, before the term 'migraine' be applied, then the condition is much less common. It would seem reasonable to include but one factor in addition to the headache, and this should be the relief of the pain by ergot.

When the life history of a migraine subject is studied, it may be observed that the accompanying features vary at different ages. So-called 'cyclical vomiting' in childhood evolves into 'bilious attacks' of adolescence and adult life, the ocular and other manifestations may or may not be present with the one constant feature—the headache—which usually tends to diminish in its intensity as the life span continues.

The one aetiological factor which seems irrefutable is the tendency for migraine to be a familial disease. This will be linked with the fact that, as has been described, the migraine patient is particularly liable to stress, and it is the latter feature that may be inherited, both genetically and environmentally. Thus the subject from a 'nervous' family, with his unresolved, usually unconscious conflicts, may find in migraine a **modus vivendi**. He might equally present his doctor with overt anxiety, depressions, or other psychosomatic conditions such as asthma, duodenal ulcer, or colitis.

There is evidence which has been presented in detail that the concept of allergy, at least in the classical sense, should not be applied to migraine. The tendency to gastric upsets which occur with the headache may have led to the erroneous conclusion that food is connected with the production of an attack.

Though the condition is commoner in women, its occurrence in men eliminates menstrual factors as being truly fundamental. In this context, the place of diuretics is of interest. It has been noted that an osmotic diuretic, urea, may be useful in the prevention of attacks. Being a physiological substance it can be given freely without fear of toxicity, but more experience of it, and particularly its evaluation in a controlled trial, are necessary before its place in treatment is settled.

The mechanics of the attack itself have been shown conclusively to be due to changes in the calibre of the intracerebral vessels. It is possible that, in addition, the latter may produce an exudate containing substances which lower the threshold to pain, though the evidence for this is far from conclusive, both experimentally and so far as treatment based upon this hypothesis is concerned.

We may say, in summary, that given a 'migraine constitution' or appropriate family background, a subject may develop attacks of headache in response to psychic factors or to physical ones such as fatigue or premenstrual hydration of the blood. A chain reaction may thus be set off consisting of a change in the calibre of (especially) certain intracranial arteries, and also possibly of other body blood vessels. It has been noted how this concept may apply to the skin, and one may postulate a wider affect if the process extends to the hypothalamus, with secondary effects upon the adrenals. Thus, features such as sweating, nausea, hypoglycaemia, and eosinopenia could be explained.

Much can be attained with regard to treatment. The attacks themselves may be cut short with drugs, and a relationship can be cultivated between the patient and his medical adviser, so that the former may understand that although he cannot change his antecedents, he can be helped to avoid situations which tend by virtue of previous associations to trigger off attacks.

Management of the patient with migraine

(1) *Between attacks*   It is suggested that patients having recurrent attacks of migraine may be more than usually the subjects of unconscious emotional conflicts and that their headaches may represent a workable, albeit unpleasant compromise. Thus, unless there is a radical resolution of these conflicts, with some regime such as extensive psychotherapy, the patient, with or without the aid of his general

practitioner, should recognise the situations in his life which may trigger off unconscious memories of conflicts and thus headaches; these situations whenever possible should be avoided. As with many psychosomatic diseases, the episodic timing, alternating with periods of normal health, make the disease the arena of every possible 'healer', from the friend with good advice, the nature curer and acupuncturist, as well as the more orthodox measures meted out by the general practitioner and hospital specialist.

In recent years, there has been an increasing appreciation of the emotional content of all illnesses, both organic and non-organic, and the medical and nursing professions are fortunately taking this aspect of disease more and more into account. Various surveys in general practice suggest that the amount of emotional illnesses diagnosed ranges from 10 to 15 per cent. It is almost certainly dependent upon the personal inclinations of the practitioner. Those who are unaware of, or loth to recognise psychological difficulties in themselves will tend to see their patients' illnesses as mostly organic, while others, with perhaps an excessive interest in the psyche and inclined naturally to introspection, will go to the other extreme and find a common denominator of anxiety in every patient. Ideally the doctor will maintain an attitude between these two excesses.

With regard to migraine, which is, *par excellence*, a general practice disease, the most significant factor in the management of the patient between attacks is the rapport and relationship between the two individuals—the patient and the doctor or nurse. The former, as a result of both recognised and unconscious difficulties in interpersonal relationships, may well be following an existence of sustained tension and anxiety.

It can be explained to the patient that tension and thus migraine may occur in two ways; either as a result of a real life difficulty, for example the necessity of relating to a difficult spouse or foreman, or as a result of a situation, in itself seemingly innocuous, but which may be unconsciously associated with a guilt or anxiety-provoking situation originally encountered perhaps many years previously. These long-forgotten events are frequently bound up with early relationships to the parents or siblings, and may be of an infantile sexual nature. Thus by association it may happen that the headaches are used as an excuse mechanism to avoid unpleasant duties or situations, such as marital relationships, with a tangible awareness of, for example, impotence or frigidity.

The basic factor here is the original conflict causing the sexual difficulties, the migraine being a 'secondary gain' in the form of a flight from the conflict. Even without the direct confrontation of the sexual situation, the headaches may save the patient from facing the guilt invoked by ambivalent feelings towards loved ones.

Out of such a discussion with the patient, it may be apparent that the migraine is, for the time being at least, the patient's best solution, as socio-economic factors may preclude radical changes in the environment, such as divorce or change of occupation. It can also be pointed out that as the patient gets older his headaches will tend to **improve**.

The knowledge that his personal doctor is aware of his difficulties, both in himself and with regard to his interpersonal relationships, will provide for the patient, perhaps for the first time, a 'good' experience, with a resulting diminution in tension. Naturally, the more intractable and severe disorders of personality require specialised treatment.

The general practitioner may reinforce the strength of the relationship, of which he is a part, by prescribing placebos and/or sedatives such as diazepam, or chlordiazepoxide.

Non-psychological measures between attacks include the administration of a ketogenic diet, this being a high-fat and low-carbohydrate regime given for a period of months. The rationale is that an alkalosis is frequently noted before the headaches, and a 'natural' acidosis is produced by voluntary fasting during the attacks.

Lastly, surgery may very occasionally be considered, the procedure usually consisting of section of selected branches of intracranial and middle meningeal arteries and their nervi vasorum.

(2) *Treatment of the attacks* Most patients will discover for themselves measures which will bring relief. Lying down in a darkened room and the self-administration of such household remedies as aspirin and sweetened drinks as well as anti-emetics, for example metoclopramide, are often used. Other analgesics, such as codeine or paracetamol, may be found by individual patients to be more efficacious than aspirin. Only in very rare instances should more powerful pain-killing preparations be necessary.

Specific Drugs—under this heading can be grouped:
(a) Antimechanical
(b) Antichemical
(c) Diuretics

Antimechanical This group consists of derivatives of the most consistently successful drug in the treatment of migraine—**ergot**. Its symptomatic success has been unsurpassed for nearly 30 years.

Ergot was first used in 1883 for the treatment of migraine, using injections of the substance in 5 cases of the disease. The first report of the drug being given by mouth was in the United States by Thomson in 1894. He also suggested the use of the drug rectally on account of the vomiting which often accompanied the headache.

A classic textbook on head pain, written by Campbell in 1894, also mentions the use of the drug. As a result of the relative impurity of the crude extracts of ergot then available, the effects produced at that time, though beneficial, were relatively inconstant, and unpredictable side-effects were often noted. Thus a refractory period with regard to its use in migraine followed until 1918, when Stoll isolated the new pure ergot alkaloid which was given the name **ergotamine**. It is interesting to note that this new preparation was first used in obstetrics and gynaecology, the characteristic action of ergot being its effect—increasing strength of contraction and muscle tone—on the pregnant uterus. In 1926, however, a French neurologist, Maiet, used the drug in the treatment of migraine.

Ergotamine, together with other related active principles, is synthesised by the ergot fungus, *Claviceps purpurea*. Ergot alkaloids are derived from lysergic acid, an indole compound which contains the characteristic indole ring structure.

The activity of the drug may be either central, affecting respiration, pulse rate and blood pressure, or peripheral. It is in this latter respect that the use of ergot in migraine is utilised. Direct stimulation of the smooth muscle in blood vessels occurs, apparently selectively, in that the maximal activity in this respect is in the walls of the intracranial arteries. **It is the most successful specific treatment for the disease.**

Administration and dosage: Ergotamine tartrate may be given by mouth, per rectum, and by injection, and an aerosol preparation has been evolved which makes it possible for the drug to be inhaled. Orally, 1 mg of ergotamine may be given at the first sign of an attack, and the dose repeated hourly for up to 6 hours.

For parenteral administration 0.25 mg subcutaneously is usually sufficient, though this may also be repeated after 4 hours. Suppositories are particularly useful when the migraine is associated with abdominal pain and vomiting. Two or three, containing 2 mg of ergotamine tartrate, may be given during any one attack. In the event of there being an indifferent response to ergotamine, dihydroergotamine may be given. This drug has a lesser vasoconstrictive activity than ergotamine, and must be given in double the dose of the latter drug. It is only effective when given by injection, the usual dose being 1–2 mg subcutaneously.

Whichever route of administration, ergot will exercise its maximum effect if the patient rests, preferably lying down, after receiving the drug.

Contra-indications to ergotamine: The drug should not be given to patients who have functional or organic disease of the blood vessels. Thus a history of angina pectoris, intermittent claudication, or overt evidence of peripheral vascular disease will preclude ergotamine therapy. Because of its effects upon the uterus, the drug should not be given during pregnancy.

Toxic Effects: The substance can itself cause headache, due to the rebound vasodilatation occurring as the effects of the drug are diminishing. A low tolerance may produce leg cramps, abdominal pain, nausea and vomiting, while, more seriously, retrosternal pain, aching in the legs, and disturbances in the heart rate or rhythm will necessitate discontinuance of the drug. The combination of ergotamine with other substances such as antihistamines, caffeine, or an atropine preparation may mitigate against these effects.

Antichemical One of the drugs used in this category is **methysergide**. In Great Britain, this drug is marketed under the name of Deseril, and in America as Sansert. The drug is a serotonin antagonist, and the basis of its use, is that there is some evidence that serotonin plays a part in the production of the migraine attack. The drug is given only prophylactically. Once an attack is established, methysergide has no place in the treatment. The dose is 1 mg 6-hourly.

Toxic Effects: Vomiting, vertigo, and leg cramps occur frequently, limiting the use of the drug to the occasional patient with severe migraine in whom other more benign remedies have failed. An occasional hazard, which has been described when administration has lasted more than three months, is **retroperitoneal fibrosis**.

Thus, though it may be worth ascertaining the effects of methysergide on patients resistant to ergot, toxic reactions should be carefully watched for, and the patients warned about them.

4 Affects

As has been reiterated in this book, the 'choice' of psychosomatic
disorder is generally determined by genetic constitution, which means
that particular individuals, and often particular families, 'break down'
in one body system rather than another and it is largely a matter of
choice of family tree. Certain factors are important in any disease but
the following points should be borne in mind especially in dealing with
a psychosomatic condition.

FAMILY BACKGROUND

As has been suggested above there will often be a record of the disease
under consideration occurring in the patient's antecedents and relatives.

DURATION

Most of the conditions described in this book occur in episodes and
tend to improve with or without treatment. The patient himself will,
according to his emotional stability, gradually come to be his own best
physician.

EARLY LIFE

Adverse situations in the environment such as death of a parent,
separation, quarrelling, cruelty and drunkenness, poverty and over-
crowding will increase the tendency to confusion in the baby and
infant's mind, the 'best' solution to which may be a psychosomatic
disease lasting throughout life.

TRAITS FOUND IN CHILDHOOD

Phenomena such as shyness, stammering, self-consciousness and blushing will highlight a personality who has found this particular method of character development a 'workable' solution to early different experiences.

WORK RECORD

Consistency and perseverence in a career is often a pointer to a person's ability to deal with life in a positive way as repeated discontent with a working situation and frequent changing of jobs is usually an effect of blaming the outside world for factors inside the patient which are too difficult for him to resolve and cope with.

SOCIAL RELATIONSHIPS

These are a particularly accurate barometer of a person's ability to effect a compromise between his own internal and emotional problems and the reality of life, as the greatest test of maturity lies in the ability of adaptation and compromise to other people. Friendships, sex, marriage and parenthood will at the deepest level indicate how satisfactorily a person has come to terms with the greatest of life's problems.

PREVIOUS ILLNESS

All G.P.s know that 90 per cent of their work is provided by 10 per cent of their patients. This means that such people by and large convert unresolved difficulties, peculiar to themselves, into what is for them a realistic reason to visit the doctor. It is usual for such people who should by no means be thought of as 'weak', inadequate or malingering, to exhibit, from time to time, disabilities and illnesses referred to most of the body systems.

The family R. The mother had died at the age of 97 after 40 years of widowhood, having reared 9 children, 7 girls and 2 boys. One boy had died relatively young, another 'disappeared' during the First World War. There was reason to believe that he had not been killed but had just decided to live abroad. Of the 7 girls, 4 never married, 1 married a first cousin late in life, another married but was childless and the last married, having one son, so of all the 9 offspring only one of them produced progeny. When grown up

36

all the girls lived within walking distance of each other and maintained consistent mutual helpful attitudes. Rowing was almost unknown and never bitter. They cared for each other, did each other's shopping and often went on holiday together. Over a period of 30 to 40 years there was never a time when at least one member of the family did not have a physical disease or accident of a moderate or severe degree. They were likeable and always pleasant and polite and the G.P. somehow never found caring for them irksome, although he was never for long not in attendance. This family illustrates how it is possible for aggression and rivalries to be denied at conscious level thus avoiding overt anger and hostility, and how such conflicts may be converted into body diseases. Among those suffered in this family were:

> *'Indigestion'*
> *Accidents involving every part of the body, including many fractures.*
> *Arthritis*
> *Constant minor infections*
> *Coronary disease and hypertension on the part of the two male spouses.*
> *Migraine*
> *Ill-defined states of fatigue, biliousness, etc.*

RECENT STRESS

It is common experience that all life crises such as bereavement, marriage, divorce, the advent of children, change of occupation and moving house may precipitate body disorders and psychological illness of all kinds.

Mrs J., moved with her husband from a small two-bedroom house to a detached four-bedroom one as a result of her husband's promotion and relatively sudden increase in income. Far from being overjoyed she immediately developed a recurrence of severe migraine lasting intermittently for several weeks. It emerged that giving up a small, known, cosy environment to which she had been used for more salubrious surroundings made her feel guilty and lost, almost as if the little house represented the most of what she felt she deserved in life (it was similar to the premises in which her own mother had brought her up). Her new prosperity somehow made her feel guilty and represented in a strange way, overtaking her own mother's fortunes.

37

VERBAL AND NON-VERBAL COMMUNICATIONS

When a person is ill the particular malady may exhibit itself in general terms, lassitude, temperature, or in more specific ways, for example pain located in an organ, difficulty in walking, loss of vision, skin rash, etc. and the doctor or nurse will piece together the patient's **symptoms** and what is discovered on examination of the patient, that is the clinical **signs**.

Mr M.Z., aged 38. This physicist noticed that after physical exertion he became hot and flushed, a normal state of events, but thought that similar sensations occurred when he was anxious or upset. As an experiment he began taking his own temperature at different times and discovered a rise of up to 2 degrees whenever professional or social events coincided with situations of anxiety for him. For example, when a confrontation with his immediate superior resulted in an open row, his temperature became 99.9 and on another occasion when sitting in a train which was delayed and resulted in him being late for an important appointment, he again discovered a pyrexia of the same extent. Subsequent similar situations were found to evoke the same response.

Appropriate investigations of the blood and urine, together with X-rays where indicated, will result in a **probable** diagnosis which is made in the form of a label, 'There is a duodenal ulcer in bed No. 4', or 'The haemophegia at the end of the ward needs a bedpan'. Naturally, what is really meant is that Mr R. C. aged 45, who has recently suffered widowhood and is struggling to maintain four teenage children, has broken down with a duodenal ulcer and Miss M. V. having cared for her elderly parents is now aged 64, and finding herself alone in the world has suffered a slight stroke. You will find very few categorical statements in this book, but one which may be applied in medical and nursing practice is that no two patients are ever exactly alike: each brings his or her own background of genetic constitution, baby, infant and grown-up experiences, family influences and the effects of 'chance' into their life pattern. Any student nurse or doctor with moderate sensitivity will perceive 'signals' from the patient which will enable a more complete diagnosis than the usual 'appendicitis', 'pneumonia', 'asthma', etc. to be made. The way the patient walks, sits or lies in bed; the resting expression; the way in which the symptoms are spoken about, whether they seem to be exaggerated or unduly minimised, and above all how the physician or nurse himself feels when he is relating to the patient. In a recent research project 'The Unpopular Patient', the many and varied attitudes to patients by nurses were found tabulated and discussed (see Further Reading).

Above all it must be understood that all symptoms, especially those found in psychosomatic diseases, are attempts by the patient to **communicate** or **manipulate his environment** or to effect a compromise solution of an unresolved, often unconscious problem; that is an attempt to effect a 'bargain'.

PSYCHOSOMATIC DISEASE AS PART OF PSYCHOSIS OR DEPRESSION

In some psychoses, particularly the type of gradual-onset schizophrenia affecting adolescents, psychosomatic disease or more correctly **hypochondriasis** may be the presenting picture. The young person will feel that first one organ then another is the seat of disorder, and the G.P. may not at first suspect the true nature of the condition.

Similarly body symptoms, again best termed 'hypochondriasis', will very frequently be part of a **depressive illness**. This refers not to the occasional miserable mood common to everyone, but a highly specific condition, the main features of which are sleep disturbance, particularly early morning wakening, anorexia, constipation and diminished libido. These attacks of depression, often called 'endogenous' to distinguish them from 'reactive depressions' which are appropriate to a life event, are usually self-limiting, but can be potentially dangerous states, due to the risk of suicide and are best treated by specialists. This **hypochondria**, often of a delusional quality (for example my "bowels are rotting away") is often found, especially if the depression is in an elderly person.

5 Somatopsychic Conditions, Overdosages and Intensive Care

It is well recognised that while emotions produce bodily symptoms, the converse is equally true, that is body illness, injury, disfigurement and operations will lead to various moods and feelings as diverse as there are various types of differing personalities. While all body malfunctions will result in some emotional and mental consequences, some conditions are particularly prone to produce overt psychiatric symptoms.

Delirium for instance, from whatever cause, implies a clouding of consciousness. This may extend from the muzzy feelings associated with fever to impairment of consciousness, a condition termed 'stupor' or 'coma'. The causes of delirium will include general disease such as that associated with the liver, the endocrine glands, infections, conditions affecting the heart and lungs, vitamin deficiencies and such as tumour, epilepsy, head injury and strokes.

FEATURES OF DEMENTIA

Memory, especially for recent events, is a particular feature which is affected. The **personality** as a whole becomes coarsened, and **intelligence** as demonstrable by simple tests, deteriorates. The patient gradually becomes careless and callous both in regard to himself and towards others. Anti-social behaviour may occur so that it is often embarrassed relatives who are the first to complain.

Dementia unlike delirium implies a gradual decline in personality, intelligence and memory, and important causes include:

Traumatic—birth injuries, head injuries
Metabolic—vitamin deficiencies, diabetes, myxoedema

40

Heredity—Huntington's Chorea
Neoplastic—tumours, especially of the bronchi and the brain
Strokes—that is cerebro-vascular disease
Degenerative—conditions of the brain, especially senile states
Infection—associated with meningitis and encephalitis

As has been said, dementia usually has a slow onset and is relatively uninfluenced by treatment. The early clinical features vary from patient to patient, and often predominant life-long personality traits in a given individual, for example meanness, irritability, suspiciousness, rapid variation in mood and depression, become accentuated at a time when the patient begins to dement.

CONDITIONS REQUIRING SURGERY

On no occasion is it so 'normal' for patients to experience fear as when they come into hospital for an operation. The illness itself which has led to the surgeon advising that an operation is necessary, the anaesthetic, the anxiety regarding pain and thoughts about the outcome and possible recurrence of the disease are all in the patient's mind; all this, in addition to the misgivings of everyone when they "go into hospital". Separation from family and friends and from an environment which to a greater or lesser extent is known and controllable is changed for one which is mostly unknown and uncontrollable. Strange figures of authority ranging from the telephonist, the hall porter, the ward orderly, all the nurses from junior probationer to matron, the ward doctors, and above all the surgeon himself come to dominate the patient's life. Usually **trust** is established in all these persons and the patient allows himself to float on the sea of expectancy and hopefulness. For many persons the anaesthetic constitutes the principal fear, as it is associated with an involuntary state of unconsciousness, that is, lack of control over oneself and the effects of oneself upon others. The anaesthetist is especially trained to deal with these fears and in modern medical practice advances in anaesthetics have been perhaps the most far-reaching of all the specialities. Extraordinary efficiency is the order of the day so that the old anaesthetic experiences such as being put to sleep by a suffocating mask, being subjected to quite toxic anaesthetic agents, and post-operative nausea and unpleasantness are nowadays virtually unknown.

It will be quite clear what a vital role the nurse can play in reassurance both before and after the actual operation. Patients vary enormously in how they express their fears: these should always be taken as present and dealt with whether they are expressed verbally or nonverbally. When the nurses seem to be confident and calm, a part of the patient's mind will **echo** this confidence and calmness to a greater or lesser extent, and autonomic effects which may seriously influence, especially, the heart and blood pressure will be reduced thus making the task of both surgeon and anaesthetist easier and indirectly considerably reducing the chances of an unsatisfactory or even fatal outcome of any particular operation. It should be remembered that the surgeon will represent the epitome of power: a figure of god-like omnipotence and where possible such confidence should be further engendered, as in the world of anasethetics and surgery it is right that regression on the part of the patient be encouraged as he is in no position to influence (once he is anaesthetised) the outcome of his operation. It is his attitude **before** the operation which can affect both the operation and post-operation phenomena: attitudes which may be considerably modified by the nursing staff. It hardly need be stated that certain operations will have special meanings and effects, examples being mastectomy and other amputations as well as the construction of colostomies and similar internal procedures, while the effects of cosmetic surgery will have repercussions of quite a different nature.

OVERDOSAGES

Over the past 10 years there has been an unprecedented rise in the incidence of **overdosages** and other gestures of self-destruction, especially wrist cutting, to the extent that nearly all General Hospitals admit daily, via their Casualty Department, a significant number of, usually, young women with this problem. **It is truly a modern epidemic,** and the attitude of the nurse whether she be on duty in the Casualty Department or in a general ward, may well be different toward such patients, compared to that she shows to others. After all, to say the least they have themselves unwittingly added to the work load of the hospital and engendered into society feelings of anxiety, frustration, irritability as well as the natural response of compassion and curiosity as to why such an event took place. (The subject is often an attractive person from a middle-class background with little overt cause to perpetrate such an act.) They are usually suffering from what psychiatrists call a personality disorder. The act itself often represents a call for help rather than a serious attempt at suicide, and is almost always part of an emotional state comprising anger and frustration, feelings which become 'transferred' to and experienced by medical and nursing staff when the latter begin to relate to the patient. The doctor usually recommends either early discharge or transfer to a psychiatric unit, partly so that the blocking of a precious bed is not perpetuated, but also because these patients are often 'unpopular', that is they do not easily provide the medical or nursing staff with professionally fulfilling experiences. These patients may not be grateful, and their personalities are often sullen, confused or overtly aggressive, the mutilating or overdosage action which brought them into hospital, being so often a thinly veiled act of hostility to someone close.

INTENSIVE CARE

A relatively recent and important hospital service is the **Intensive Care Unit** and it is here that somatopsychic phenomena are particularly demonstrable. Apart from the patients in these units, those nursing them are also often shown to be particularly vulnerable to the stress, of what is after all a literally life and death setting surrounded by highly sophisticated monitoring and therapeutic apparatus. These units are now well established in most modern hospitals and patients suffering from a variety of conditions ranging from coronary disease, polyneuritis, post-cardiac surgery and respiratory failure from many causes, will be nursed there. Apart from the appropriate anxiety felt by all, it has been found that a simple apathetic depression often occurs in the patients, surprisingly enough after the acute crisis situation has been resolved, so that they become silent and uncooperative and need firm handling by their attendants. The condition usually resolves within a few days. A very frightening experience for any patient who has been on a ventilator, occurs when the apparatus is removed, as fear and anxiety about suffocating, especially in the night, are particularly common.

Tomlin, in his article 'The Stress of the Nursing Staff' (*British Medical Journal*, **2**, 1977 (441–443)), highlights the stress on the nursing staff who are in charge of these units. He says:

Nurses who staff such units are among the elite of their profession. The level of clinical responsibility that they have to exercise is extremely high. If they are to feel secure in their professional judgment the academic knowledge they need to have to understand what is happening to their patients—and to interpret any changes they observe—is also very substantial. For optimum patient care it is better for the same nurse to look after the same patient for each shift they are on duty. They then get to know their patients and their individual foibles extremely well and can elicit, by persistent persuasion, maximum co-operation and effort from the patient, whether this is to cope with the patient's sagging morale or clear the chest of retained secretions. Yet the mortality of the patients is high. All this imposes severe demands on the staff and when, despite a lot of hard work and effort, death occurs unexpectedly they can be greatly disturbed by it.

As a result of the stresses of working in an intensive care unit at least three nurses working in different intensive care units have taken or attempted to take their own lives. Two succeeded, and in both cases the precipitating circumstances were identical. A patient apparently near recovery, whom the nurse had looked after for a long time, died unexpectedly and in rather dramatic circumstances while the nurse was present. One patient died from a massive secondary haemorrhage from an aortic graft and the other, a young severe chronic asthmatic, died while inhaling isoprenaline. Both nurses took drugs and other equipment (syringes, cannulas, etc.) from the unit and used the drugs after coming off duty. The third nurse, who was working under severe pressure in a very busy unit with several decerebrate patients, also took drugs from the unit intending to commit suicide but was found and resuscitated in time. She was subsequently treated for acute depression.

It is difficult to know how best to reduce these effects of stress on staff. Rotating staff to other parts of the hospital for periods creates dissatisfaction as they cannot use their highly prized knowledge and skills outside the intensive care unit. They therefore resign. Leadership, individual counselling, and a sympathetic nursing administration can do much to lessen the effects of this stress but do not always succeed. Holidays and extra time off when the patient work load is slack help but may cause conflict with other members of the hospital community, especially with a remote bureaucratic administration. This is particularly so when urgent requests to draft in extra staff, agency nurses, etc., are made to cope with unusual patient loads, as happens periodically. Recognition and appreciation by senior medical staff of the care that has been given to their patients is also important in mitigating the effects of this stress. Clearly, if this should prove to be a widespread problem then perhaps psychological screening of the staff may be worth considering.

While it may be as Dr Tomlin suggests, that it is the elite of the nursing profession who choose to work in and are accepted by intensive care units, there may also be other factors such as the dramatic setting of such units appealing to those of a particular disposition, and a minority of such personnel could themselves be susceptible to a breakdown as a result of the very circumstances of work that they themselves have chosen.

Further in somatopsychic considerations, we may consider how any illness of more than trivial importance, will remind the sufferer of his own vulnerability and infallibility. Feelings of helplessness, guilt, hatred and envy towards those not suffering will result in depression and anxiety, this is apart from the secondary **benefit** that being ill bestows on the patient. 'Illness' means of course that the ordinary commitments of family and society, and the confrontations with those liable to cause angry feelings, may be avoided.

6 Management

(1) Specific to the disease itself, for example Hypotensive drugs—
anti-spasmodics for asthma, ergot for migraine, etc.

(2) Non-specific measures.

(3) The special role and opportunities for the nurse, and other 'caring'
professionals:—**TRANSFERENCE**

When it has been decided, as a result of examination and investiga-
tion, that a considerable part of the total clinical picture is due to
anxiety or other emotionally determined factors, the medical and
nursing professions have at their means several alternatives and com-
binations of treatment to use. As the terms of reference of this book
are psychosomatic disease, it is not proposed to go into detail regarding
moderate or major psychiatric illnesses such as severe depression and
schizophrenia. The very fact that a patient is in hospital is frequently
therapeutic in itself as it means that society, relatives and friends have
acknowledged the person's right to receive care and help, and that he is
'worthy' for this to take place. Naturally such a formulation is never
spelt out but is implicit in the total situation of hospital admission or
even out-patient care. In the majority of conditions where a specific
event needs to be altered or cured, for example pneumonia, appendicitis,
childbirth, there will be in most cases no need for any further considerations towards the patient's mental state other than perhaps a mild
sedative at night. When, however, it has been decided that stress or
unresolved anxiety is playing a part in the maintenance of the symptoms, then notwithstanding a specific measure such as gastrectomy or
administration of anti-hypertensive drugs, those caring for the patient

may wish to use other measures, which can be divided into specific and non-specific.

SPECIFIC TO THE DISEASE

As already mentioned examples would be hypotensive drugs. Ephedrine for acute asthma, and antacids prescribed for indigestion and peptic ulcer.

NON-SPECIFIC MEASURES

Psychotropic Drugs

The past 20 to 30 years have seen significant advances in the development of groups of drugs used for both major and minor psychiatric conditions. Bromides were available in the early part of this century as a sedative, but their limited and unpredictable effects coupled with a tendency to many side-effects, especially those causing troublesome skin conditions, led to the stimulus for further, intensive research in this field: so much so that now the doctor has a bewildering choice at his disposal though psychotropic drugs have no effect on the basic cause of mental disease or personality disorders, and their therapeutic use is in controlling symptoms. Those used as an adjuvent to rehabilitation or psychotherapy have a place in the total management of many patients. In one field especially they have been a particularly significant factor in reducing in-patient care: that is with regard to psychotic subjects especially schizophrenics, wherein the drugs known as phenothiazines have established themselves. In the past five years, **lithium** also has come to have a significant place in the treatment of **manic** and **depressive states**.

The term 'psychotropic' refers to having an effect on the mental state (mood, feelings, ability to think, to conceptualise). When applied to drugs, it may be helpful to regard such substances as psycho-sedative or psycho-stimulant (see Table 1), though an exact, clear-cut, pharmacological action is not always possible as for example, by reducing depression, a drug may cause a secondary stimulation of mental activity.

The decision whether or not to use these substances lies within the province of the physician who may be a psychiatrist, but quite fre-

Table 1 Therapeutic classification of psychotropic drugs with examples of each group (based on W.H.O.)

Function	Group	Classes	Representatives
Psycho-sedatives	Neuroleptics	Reserpine type	Reserpine
		Phenothiazine type	Chlorpromazine, Chlorprothixene
		Butyro-phenones	Haloperidol
	Tranquillisers	Some phenothiazines	Promazine Flupherazine*, promethazine
		Propanediols	Meprobamate
		Hypnosedatives	Amylobarbitone, phenobarbitone
		Benzodiaze-pines	Chlordiazepoxide diazepam, nitrazepam
Psycho-stimulants		Amphetamine type	Dexamphetamine
	Euphoriants Thymoleptics	Imipramine group	Imipramine, desipramine
		Amitriptyline group	Amitriptyline, nortriptyline
	Lithium carbonate	—	Lithium carbonate
	MAOIs		Iproniazid, isocarboxazid

*Fluphenazine ('Moditen') can be given by long-acting injections every 2–3 weeks and is particularly useful in controlling schizophrenic patients who cannot be relied upon to take their drugs by mouth.

quently all doctors and especially G.P.s use them when they feel it is appropriate to do so, notwithstanding that the main reason for the patient coming to them is, say, a surgical operation or a skin irritation. In other words, more often than not, and especially in hospital, patients require additional medication in the form of, say, mild sedation and hypnotics.

Drugs in depression

Psychiatrists have found that antidepressant drugs often do away with the need for shock therapy. Such drugs include tricyclic compounds for example Tofranil and Triptizol, tetracyclic preparations for example Ludiomil, a miscellaneous group of antidepressants such as Vivalin and Optimax, and lastly the monoamine oxidase inhibitors, (MAOIs) such as Nardil and Parnate. With this group certain dietary restrictions, especially for cheese are necessary. Finally lithium is now being used to prevent recurrent attacks of mania and depression.

Psychotherapy

In the sphere of psychiatry, certain specialists do not use drugs but treat exclusively by the exchange of words with the patient. Broadly speaking such doctors may use reassurance, and here again it is not exclusively psychotherapists and physicians who are gainfully employed as such, but friends, clergymen, and many trained laymen and women, equipped to listen to, and advise people in trouble. The nurse will, of course, have a very special function in this regard because of both her medical knowledge and her close connection with the patient. There are, in addition, a special group of doctors and laymen, trained, not only to advise but also to interpret back to the patient the results of the latter's verbalisations of their problems. These **psychotherapists** include psycho-analysts (followers of Freud) and analytical psychologists (adherents of Jung). This special form of psychotherapy is highly technical, requiring a long and arduous training and such practitioners will expect to see their patients over a considerable time, as they deal mainly with severe forms of mental disturbance, though people with adequate and successful lives, but who may feel that they are getting rather bad 'bargains' in terms of their personal relationships, also constitute much of the psychoanalysts' case-load.

Hypnosis and Psychosomatic Disease

The treatment of patients by hypnosis receives considerable attention from time to time and is at present an accepted form of therapy. Its chief use is in the amelioration of symptoms and it has a particular application when a hypnotisable subject has any troublesome psycho-somatic condition. Success using hypnosis has been reported in almost every type of these illnesses, even on one classic occasion a well-documented case of pemphigus, where the patient was actually dying of this suppurative skin condition. The phenomenon of hypnosis is one where the hypnotist 'suggests' to the patient that control of his (the subject's) own emotions, and hence physical sequelae, is possible.

49

The mechanism is not understood, but works under different designations such as faith healing, and the many forms of fringe medicine techniques commonly practised. In some way, direct access to the patient's unconscious mind is reached and authoritative or permissive messages which are transmitted from the healer to the subject may result in mental or physical improvement. The drawbacks are that not all patients can be hypnotised, the essential conflict is not treated or even understood, and the effects are usually temporary. Indeed, one set of physical symptoms may abate only to become converted into another manifestation of the same unconscious unresolved conflict.

Nurse Therapists

Recently certain nurses have become trained in **behaviour therapy** a term referring to a wide variety of treatment methods designed to remove usually a single distressing clinical feature. It does not attempt to modify the personality, but is extremely useful in selected cases in dealing with the anxiety associated with especially phobias, sexual disturbances, compulsive stealing, addictions and other conditions which impose a great strain on the sufferer and his family. It has been found that it is not necessary for psychiatrists themselves to carry out the treatments which are often some form of **desensitisation**, and nowadays suitable registered mental nurses are being trained to become behavioural psychotherapists for adult neurotic disorders. The scheme is largely a success (see *Nursing Times*, **69**, September 1973, 153–156).

THE CONCEPT OF TRANSFERENCE AND THE NURSE

It is a well-known fact that we often have preconceived ideas about people before we even meet them. This is especially illustrated in the case of the child who may exhibit fear of figures of authority such as policemen. Such premature judgments are based on previous experience and feelings which we invest into early events with the very first people with whom we come in contact, usually our parents.

Clearly the concept of 'nurse' implies to all, a 'good mother' who will care, remain concerned, comfort in word and deed and 'take over' the baby, anticipating its needs and putting her own well-being behind that of the baby (patient). This ideal state may or may not occur in real infant life but its expectation in the nurse/patient relationship is invariable. We are not concerned here with what motivated a person to become a nurse, though clearly there is an invariable component of wanting to experience and thus let others experience a good mother, either one who is actually remembered from the nurse's own childhood, or just as frequently the sort of mother whom the nurse would have liked to have had as a child.

The concept of these 'transferences' that is the investment of persons 'remembered' from childhood has some disadvantages. When for instance the nurse (mother) fails to live up to expectations, she may unreasonably become changed in the patient's (child's) mind into a bad nurse/mother and experienced as such. From the earliest days in the wards caring for patients the student nurse will have the evidence of these concepts. She will be met with every kind of personality; the overtly fearful, the angry, the submissive, the flattering, the genuinely appreciative and the inveterate trouble maker. As she is only human she will probably react in a different way to each kind of 'signal'. Interestingly enough, what a particular patient makes her feel is often a clue to the diagnosis of that patient's personality. In other words, the patient can be said to 'put into the nurse' feelings which are felt by him, so that if a given patient makes a nurse feel angry she must try to understand that that particular patient probably is himself angry (at being ill, at being forced to seek help from others). She should not take it as a sign of a personal vendetta. Other patients will exhibit their fears, as has been said, in ways such as inordinate meekness, or submissiveness.

It is apparent that the nurse has the privilege of representing the ultimate in the good transference: that is, for all mankind, she can if she wishes, come to stand for the Good Mother, who is concerned, has expertise and the task of comforting. But unlike her medical colleagues, she actually handles, feeds, washes and attends to the evacuations of the patient, as well as the administering of drugs and other distress-relieving agents: a unique opportunity for fulfilment in today's materialistic society.

Further Reading

Altschul, A. *Psychology for Nurses*. 4th edn, Bailliere, London (1975)

Gillis, L.*Human Behaviour in Illness: Psychology and Interpersonal Relations*. Faber, London (1972)

Klein, M. and Riviere, J. *Love, Hate and Reparation*. Hogarth Press, London (1975)

Maxwell, H. *Integrated Medicine: The Human Approach*. John Wright, Bristol (1976)

Munro, (ed.) *Psychosomatic Medicine*. Churchill Livingstone, Edinburgh (1973).

Salzberger-Wittenberg, I. *Psychoanalytic Insights and Relationships: A Kleinian Approach*. Routledge and Kegan Paul, London (1970)

Stockwell, F. *The Unpopular Patient*. Royal College of Nurses (1972)

Index